Gage's New Friend

A Boy's Wish For A Diabetic Alert Dog

By Gage Bunsness with Kimberly Bunsness

Illustrated by Kimberly Bunsness

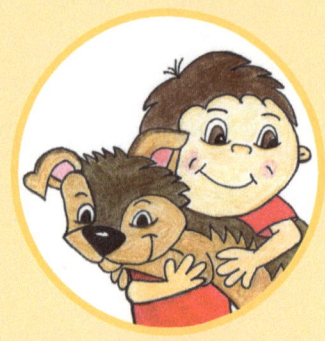

ISBN: 1482610914

ISBN 13: 9781482610918

Gage's New Friend

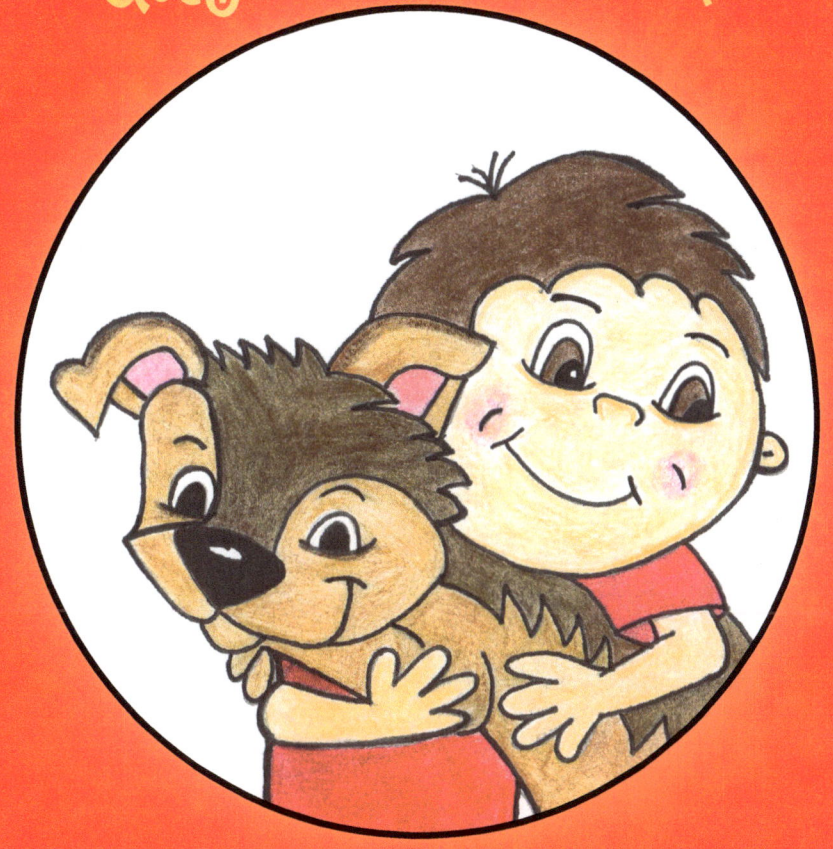

Written By Gage

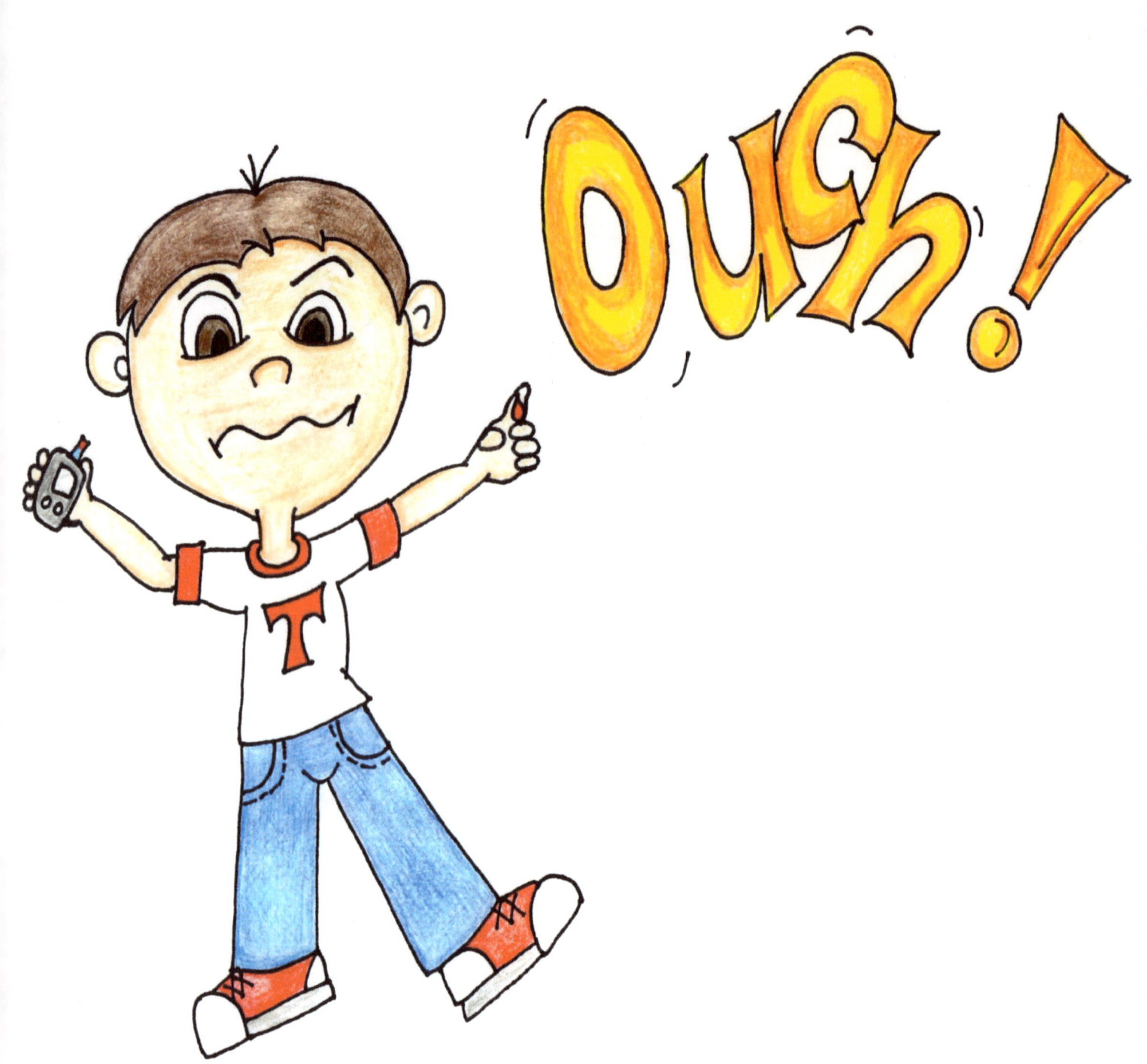

My name is Gage. I am ten-years old and I have Type 1 Diabetes. I do not like having diabetes at all. I have to test my blood sugar 10 to 12 times a day. I have to poke myself with a needle and sometimes it hurts.

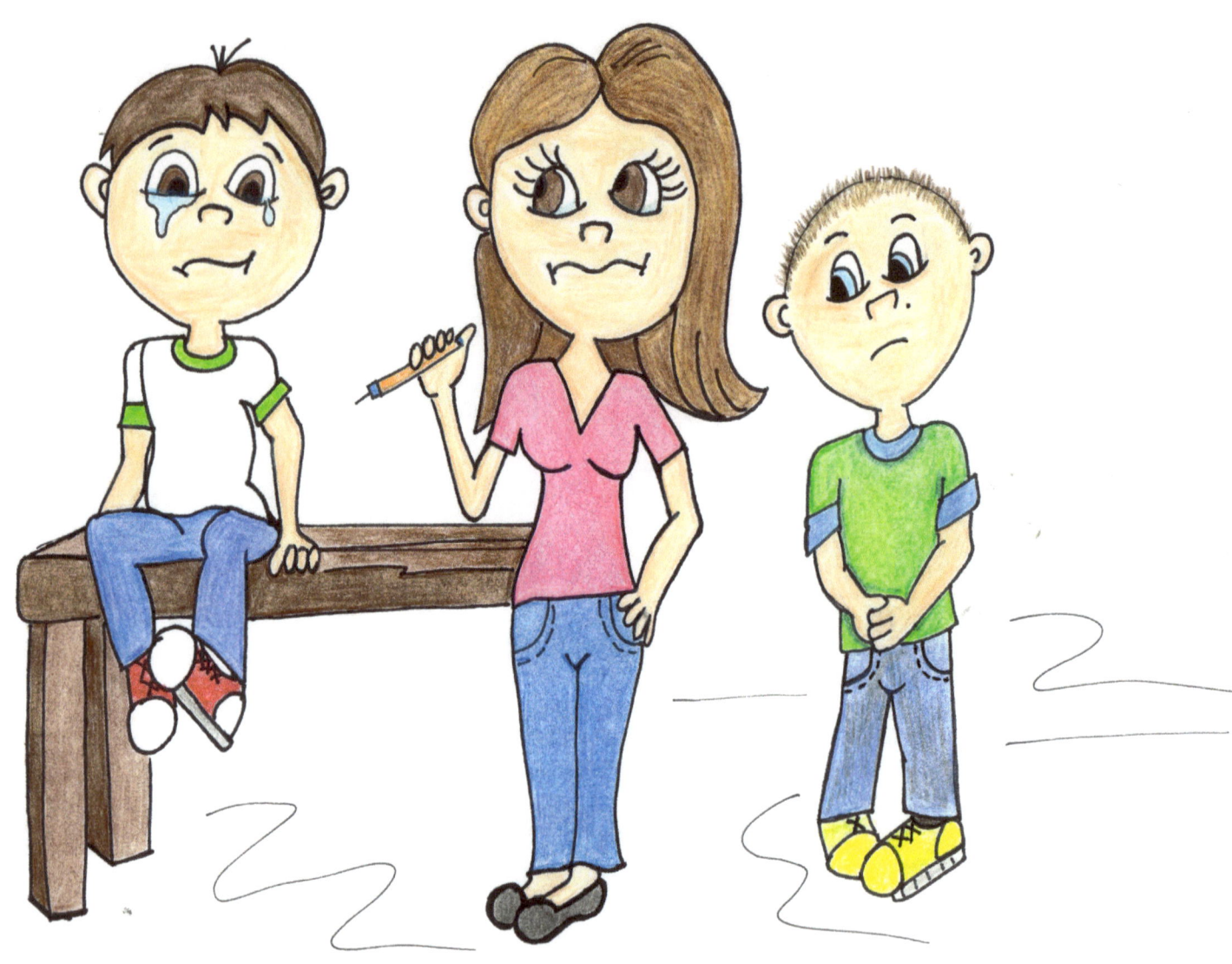

When I was first diagnosed, I had to take insulin shots. Sometimes it would make me cry. After 2 months, I got an insulin pump to deliver my insulin. It made things a little easier, but things are still hard on me.

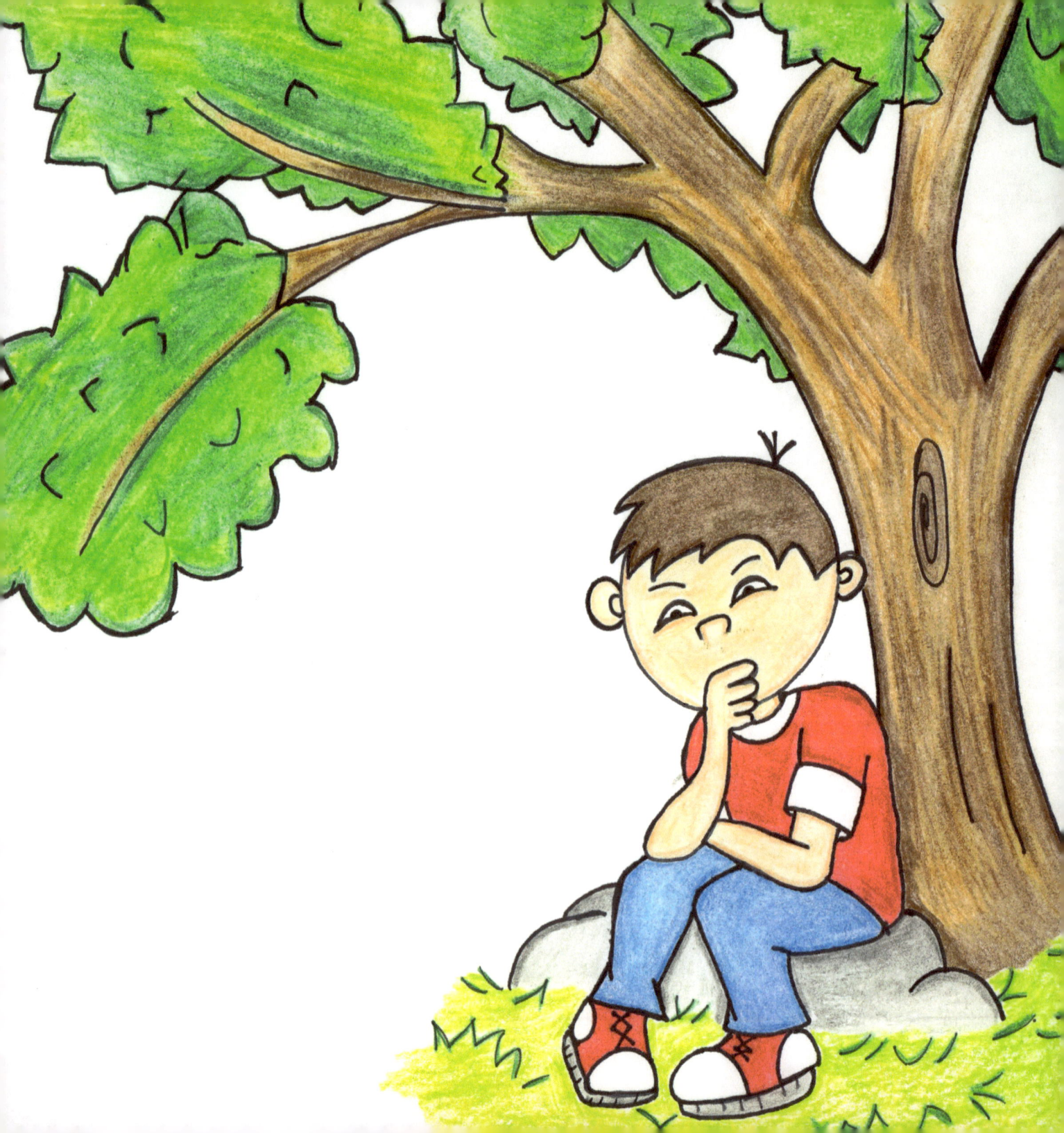

I wished for someone or something to help make my diabetes easier. One day my mom looked for someone or something to help me. She found out about Diabetic Alert Dogs, dogs that are trained to help manage diabetes. She knew a Diabetic Alert Dog would be perfect for me.

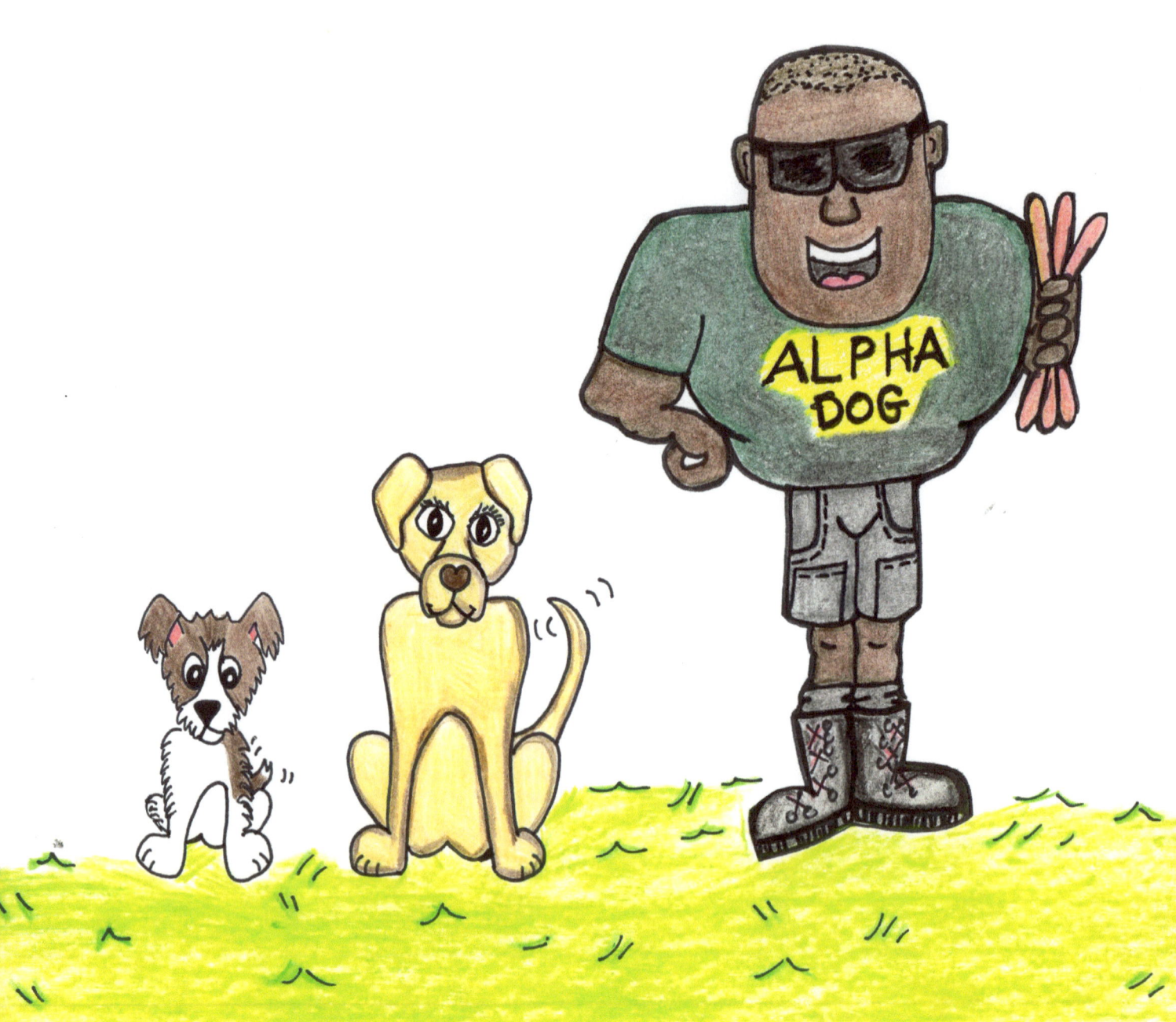

My mom was able to find a special dog trainer. The dog trainer would train a Diabetic Alert Dog for me. It would alert me when my blood sugar was going too low or too high. If I was unable to help myself, the dog would go get my mom or dad.

My mom and dad made a secret plan with the trainer to get me a Diabetic Alert Dog.

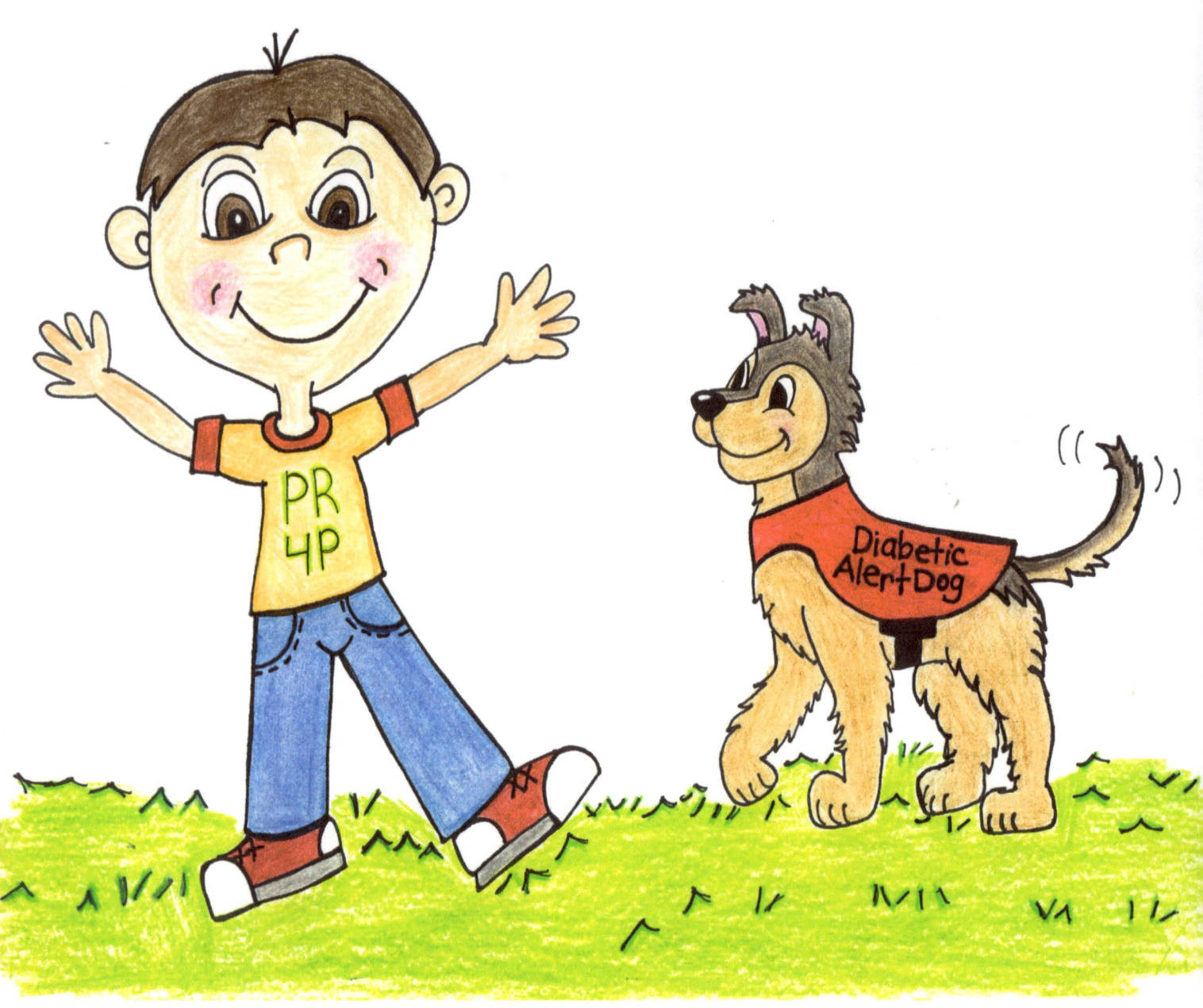

After a year, I was finally introduced to my new friend. I was so surprised and happy, I had someone to play with and help me. I named my new best friend Echo.

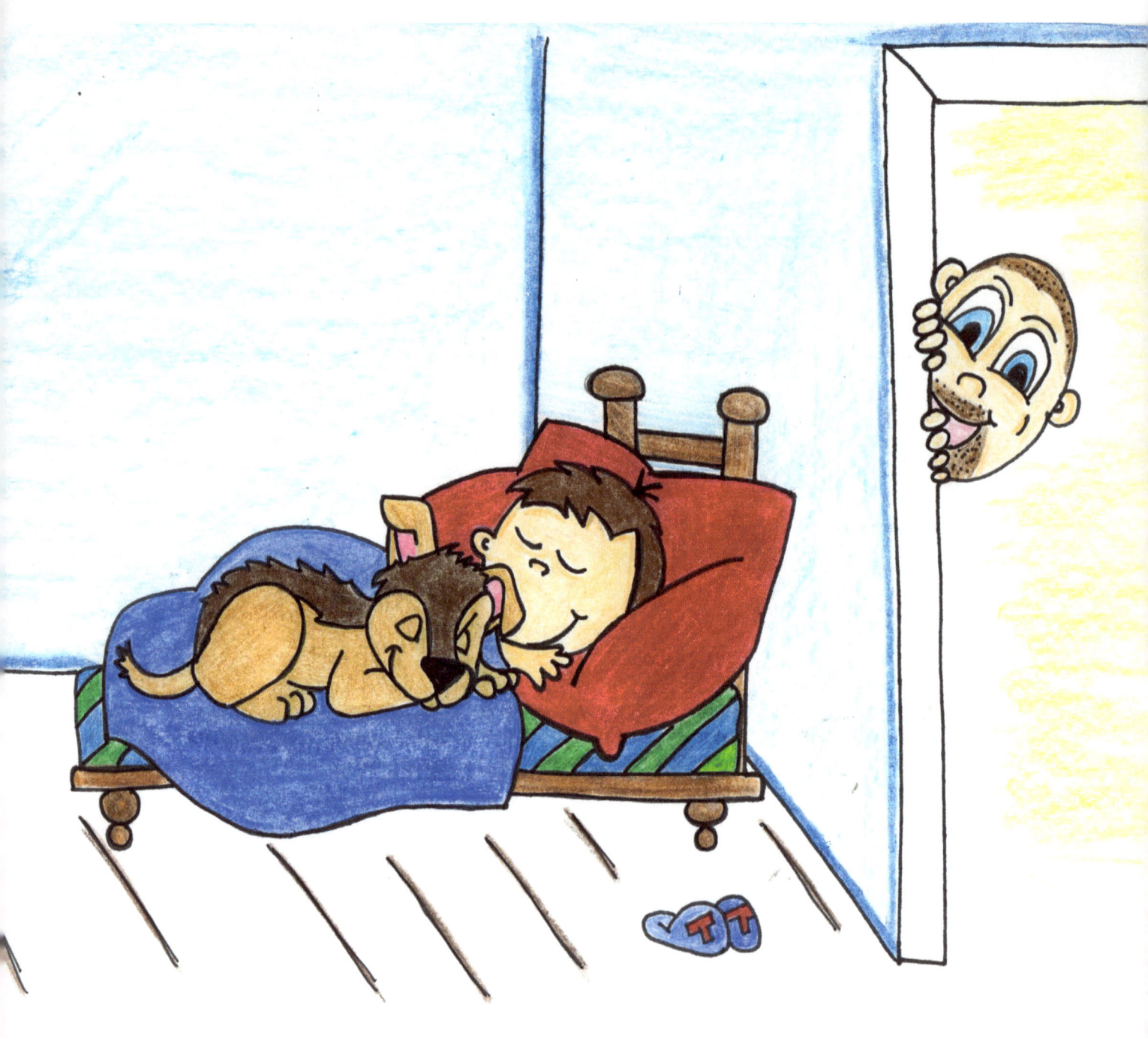

That night my new dog Echo slept with me. My mom and dad were also happy that Echo and I would have many adventures together. My parents drifted off to sleep knowing my guardian angel named Echo was looking after me.

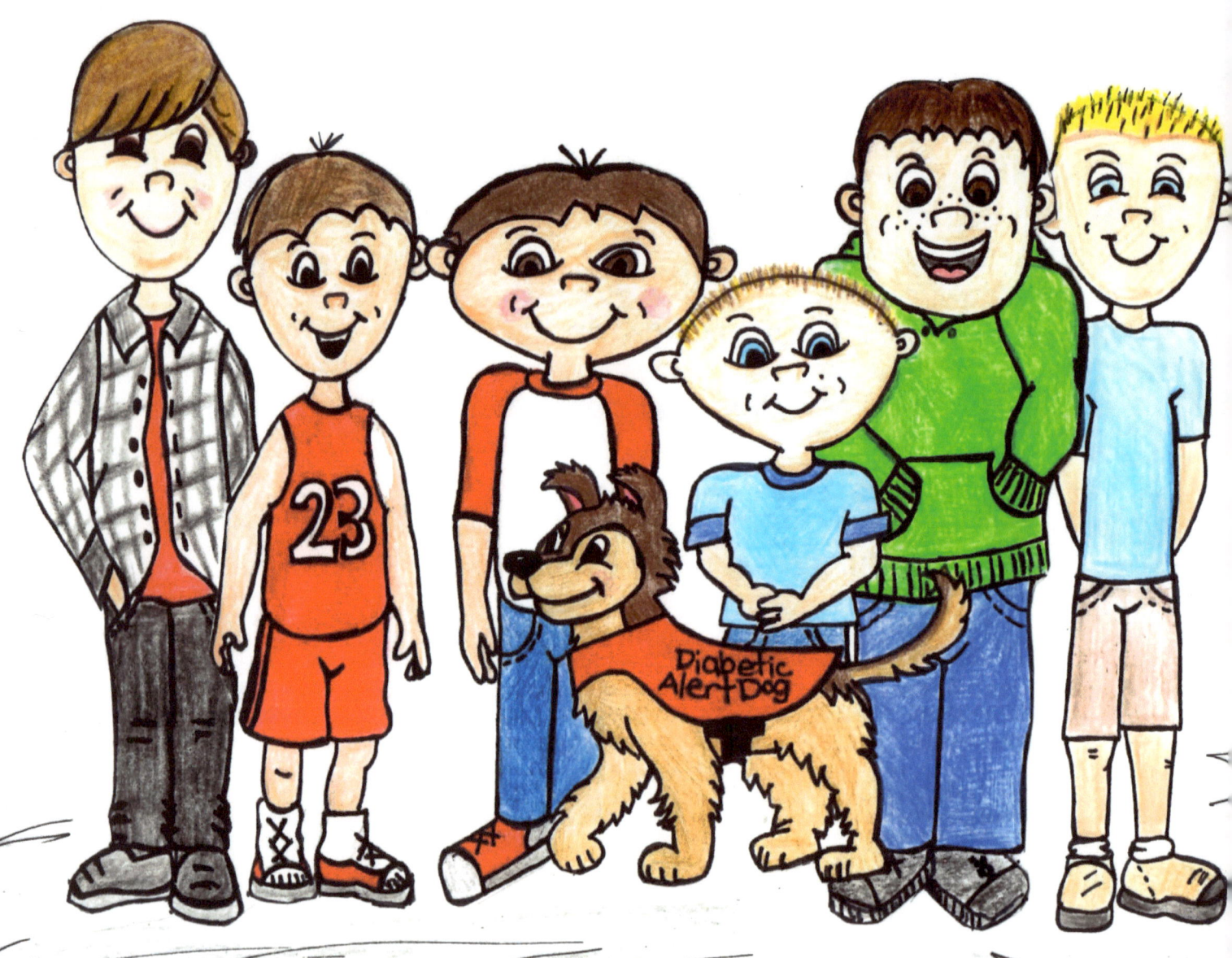

Author's Notes:

It really stinks always having to test my blood sugar and poke myself. When I get a diabetic alert dog, it will make me so happy. I can have a dog that alerts before I go low so I can have a snack and continue to play with my friends. I thank my mom, dad and brother for always being there for me and being so supportive. I also thank my friends for being kind and not thinking of me as being weird. My favorite thing to do is to be outdoors. My favorite thing to do outdoors is go camping. Kids with diabetes are just like any other kids.

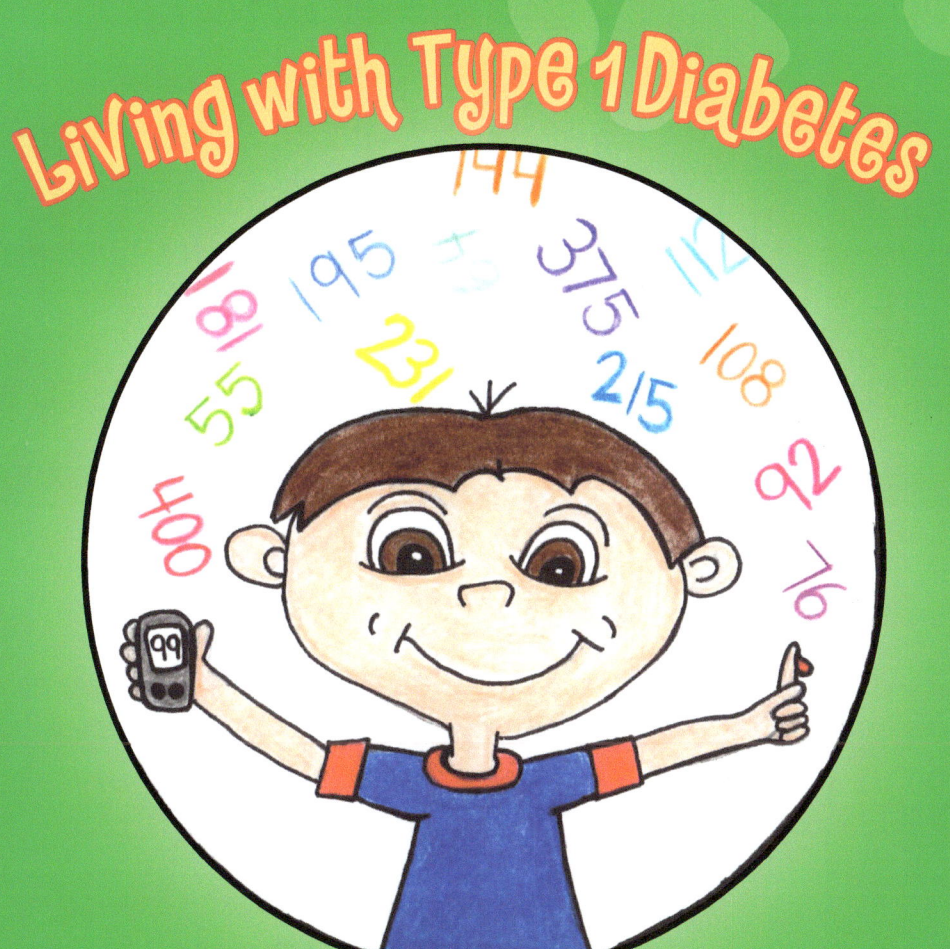

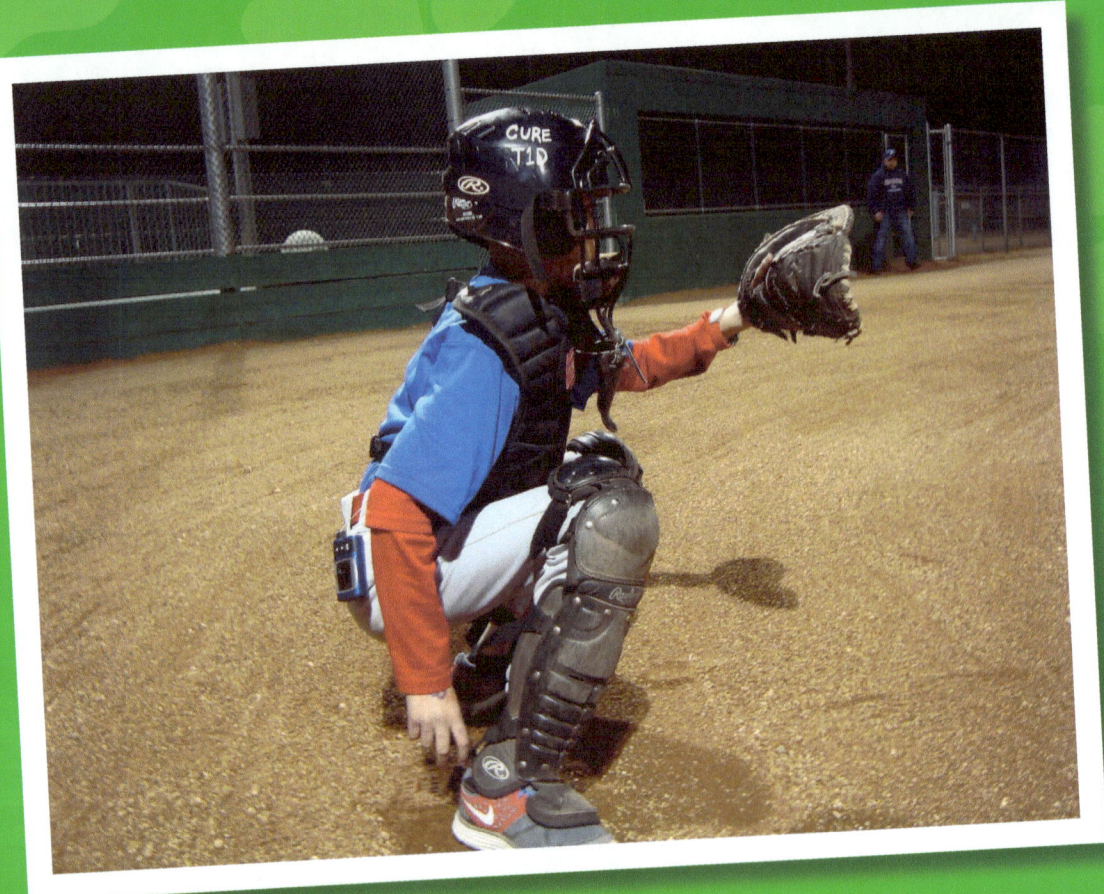

YOU CAN'T CATCH TYPE 1 DIABETES
BUT YOU CAN STILL CATCH WITH TYPE 1 DIABETES.

↗Chasing Numbers

On November 30, 2010, our son, Gage, was taken to the ER by ambulance. Shortly after arrival, he was diagnosed with Type 1 Diabetes. At the time, he was eight-years old. When he was first diagnosed, he had to take insulin shots 4-5 times every day to stay alive. He now wears an insulin pump. This is just another means to deliver insulin to the body. It does not check his blood sugar, it does not shut off when his blood sugar is too low, it does not give more insulin when his blood sugar is too high. It does what we tell it to do when we tell it to do it.

Type 1 Diabetes is also known as Juvenile Diabetes. It is an autoimmune disease. The insulin-producing cells in the pancreas stop working. Our bodies need insulin; it helps sugars pass into our cells for energy. Insulin also helps our liver to stop passing too much sugar into our blood.

Without insulin, the body will start to break down fats and muscles for energy. The broken-down fats turn into ketones. Ketones are acids. High levels of ketones are toxic to the body. This is known as DKA, which stands for Diabetic Ketoacidosis. This is a serious condition that can cause coma or even death.

In a non-diabetic child, normal blood sugar range is 70-130 in a random blood test.

My son's doctor would like his blood sugar range between 80-180.

Just like too high of blood sugar is dangerous, so is too low. Low blood sugar can also cause coma or death.

After awhile, some diabetics become unaware of their low and high blood sugars. They can no longer feel the symptoms coming on. Because of this unawareness, their lives are always at risk of falling into a coma or worse.

Gage tests his blood sugar 10-12 times a day. This is done by a finger prick. Not fun. His fingertips are sore at times and calloused. His pump is only taken off when he showers. He is pretty much attached to it 24/7. There is a small catheter under his skin connected to fine tubing that is connected to his pump. This is changed every other day.

He has to stop playing when his blood sugar drops too low. He will sit out and drink juice and watch his friends from the side. When his blood sugar is too high, he is given more insulin. He has to drink water until he feels like he can't take another sip. This is so he can pass the high levels of sugar out in his urine so he doesn't end up in DKA.

His younger brother misses having an older brother that doesn't have to worry about his blood sugar all the time. It takes away from their play time. As a mom and dad, your heart aches because you can't take it away. You can only try and make things a little easier.

Gage is now ten years old. He is a strong, brave boy that continues to live life to the fullest. He loves baseball and playing army like most boys his age. He is an amazing big brother. His heart is full of love. He is involved with helping other kids with diabetes and educating the community about Type 1 Diabetes.

Every night I set my alarm at 12:30am to check his blood sugar. My husband does the testing at 5am. Some nights we have to wake him up from his happy dreams to have him drink milk or juice because his blood sugar has dropped too low during the night. We retest in 15 minutes to make sure it is back in the safe zone. If his blood sugar is still too low we must repeat giving him juice every 15 minutes until his blood sugar is high enough to let him continuing sleeping through the night.

At this time there is no cure for diabetes. It is a constant game of chasing numbers from lows to highs. We would like to be able to be proactive rather than reactive. Our hope is for Gage to get a Diabetic Alert Dog. This is a service dog that will be able to go everywhere with him. This four-legged friend will be our eyes, ears and nose when we cannot be with him. An alert dog has the ability to let the person living with diabetes know if their blood sugar is getting too low or too high on average 30 minutes before it happens. These amazing animals are able to find help if the person is unable to help themselves. They are like angels watching over your child. These dogs cost anywhere from $20,000 - $25,000.

They are not covered by insurance.

As Gage gets older, he would like to be more independent. It is so uncool to have your mom with you all the time.

Gage's wish is to have a best friend that can help him manage his diabetes.

Know the Warning Signs So A Loved One Does Not End Up In DKA

- Frequent Urination
- Excessive Thirst
- Heavy, Labored Breathing
- Sudden Weight Loss
- Fruity, Sweet Odor to the Breath
- Sudden Vision Changes
- Sudden Bed Wetting

Type 1 Diabetes Truths:

- You CANNOT catch Type 1 Diabetes.

- Type 1 Diabetes is NOT caused from poor diet and not enough exercise!

- Type 1 Diabetes is an autoimmune disease.

- Insulin is NOT a cure. Insulin sustains life until a cure is found.

- Type 1 Diabetes CAN lead to blindness, kidney failure, neuropathy and amputation.

- Children with Type 1 Diabetes CAN still play sports, go to birthday parties, go on vacation and have sleepovers.

- People with Type 1 Diabetes CAN still eat treats: cakes, cookies, pies, ice-cream, brownies and candies; they just have to have insulin to balance it. Of course, like anyone else, it is a treat. A balanced diet is best for all children, diabetic or not.

Dog Biscuit Recipes

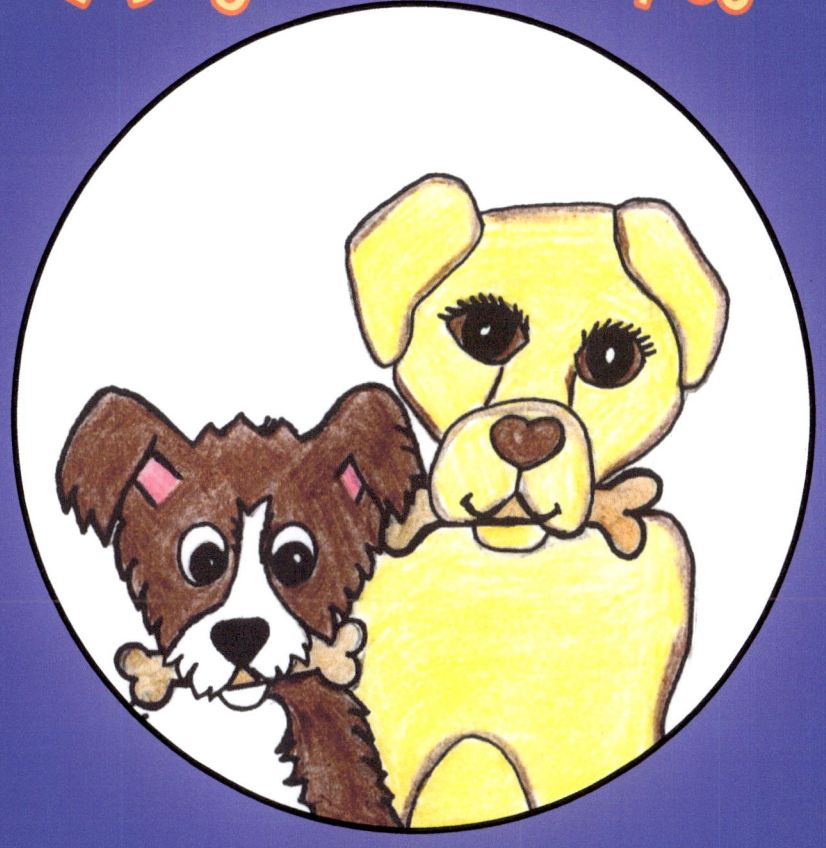

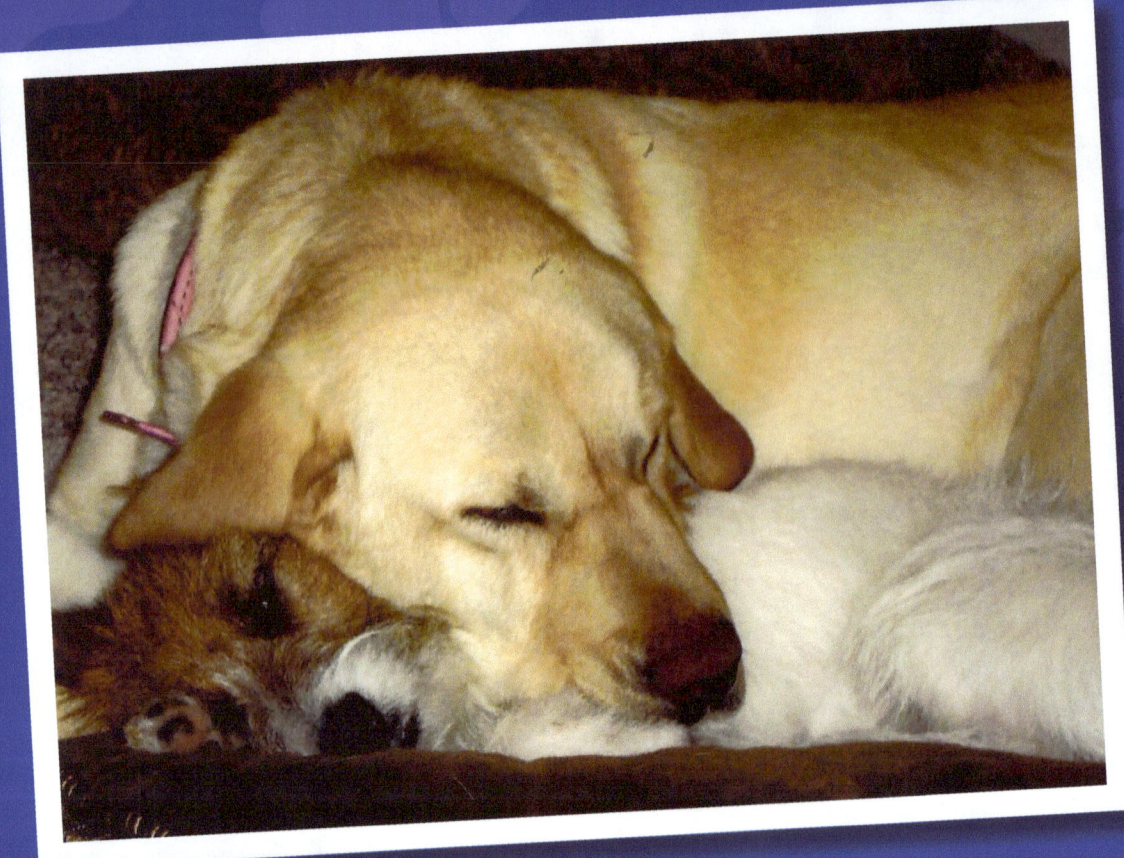

"WINNIE AND FRIDAY"

A few years ago I decided to try making a dog cookie without corn or wheat. Quickly, my first recipe, "Friday's Cookies," grew into a total of six lip-smacking treats. I have shared these cookies with friends' pets over the past few years, with always the same response: "My dogs love them!" "Can I buy some?" and "Can I have the recipe?" I have not shared my secret recipes up until now. As a thank you for your support, I have included all six original recipes. I hope you enjoy making them and your four-legged friends love them as much as ours do.

Tips:

For these recipes I use blended oats (rolled oats put in a food processor to make oat flour), natural peanut butter; if the fresh fruit is not available, I will use frozen, but always without sugar. If the dough seems too dry, I will add a little bit of water.

Thank You and Happy Baking ☺

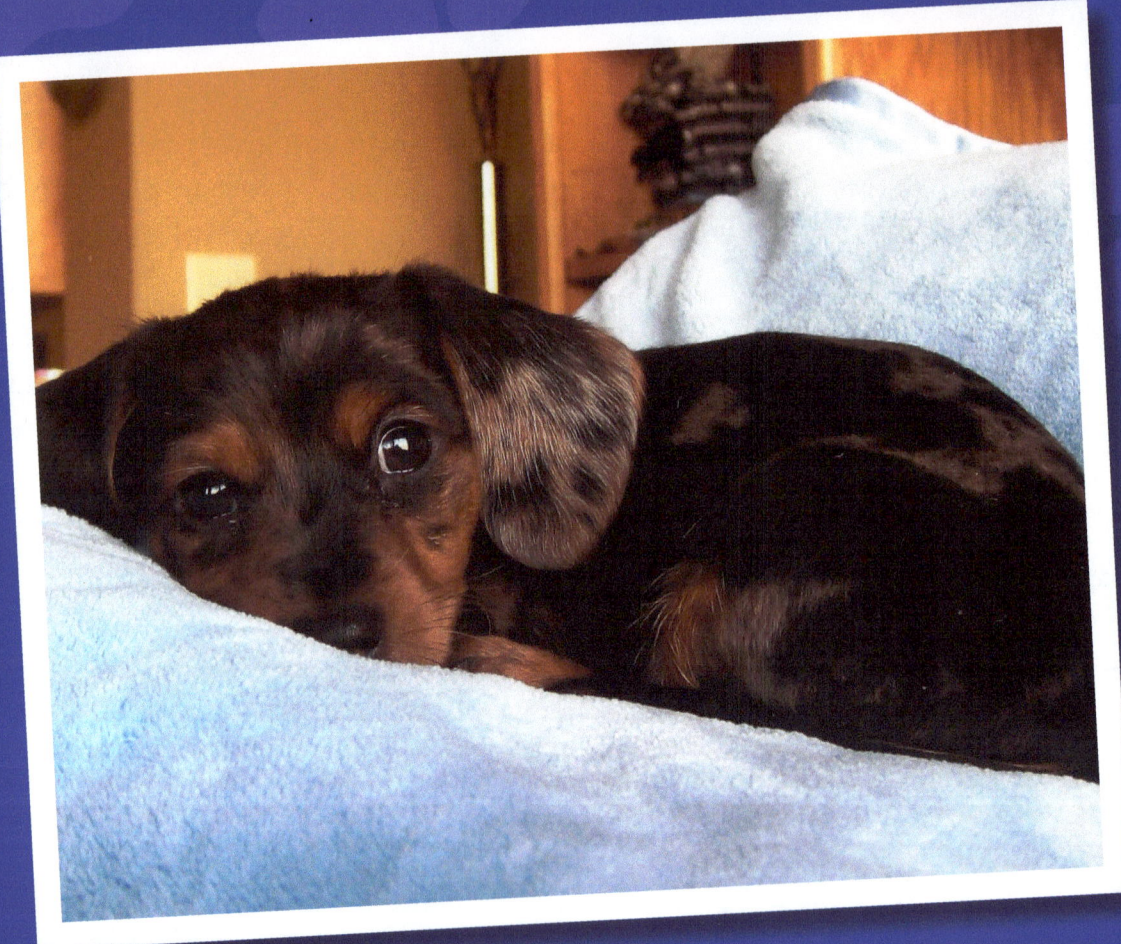

"BLITZ"

Banana-Berry Blitz
(banana/blueberry)

Bake at 400 degrees for 18-24 minutes.

In large bowl, smash bananas with a fork. Place blueberries into a blender and lightly blend; add blueberries to bananas. Put honey in microwave for 5 seconds, add to banana mixture. Next add 3 eggs. Mix by hand until well blended.

Add oats to banana mixture slowly, mix by hand. Continue to add until all oats have been mixed in.

You want the dough medium to firm.

Roll out ¼ inch thick onto oat-floured surface. Cut with your favorite cookie-cutter shapes.

Place on ungreased cookie sheet. Turn over when it has been ½ the cooking time.

Bake until golden brown.

- **2 bananas**
- **1 ½ cups blueberries**
- **2 tablespoons honey**
- **3 eggs**
- **6 cups blended oats**

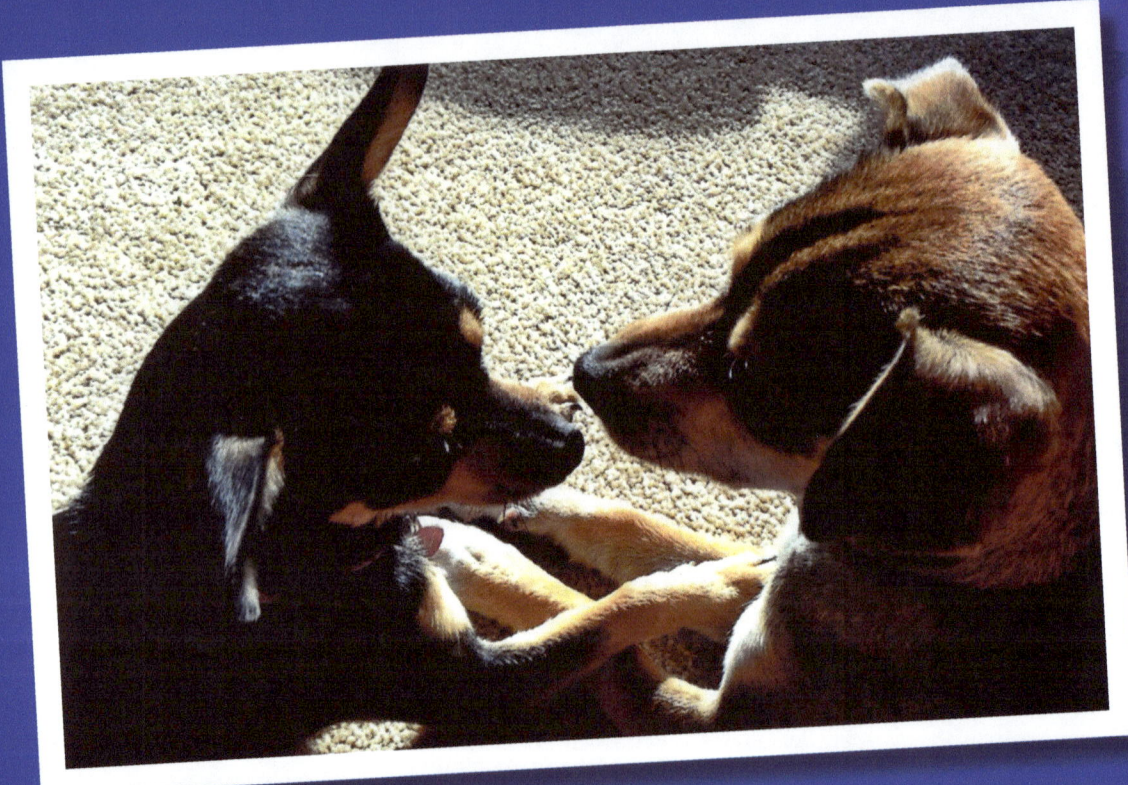

"IZZY AND NICK"

Buddy Biscuits
(pumpkin/cranberry)

Bake at 400 degrees for 18-24 minutes.

In large bowl, add pumpkin puree. Place cranberries into a blender and lightly blend; add cranberries to pumpkin. Next, add 3 eggs. Mix by hand until well blended.

Add oats to pumpkin mixture slowly, mix by hand. Continue to add until all oats have been mixed in.

You want the dough medium to firm. You do not want sticky dough.

Roll out ¼ inch thick onto oat-floured surface. Cut with your favorite cookie-cutter shapes.

Place on ungreased cookie sheet. Turn over when it has been ½ the cooking time.

Bake until golden brown.

- 1 cup pumpkin puree
- 1 ½ cups fresh cranberries
- 3 eggs
- 6 cups blended oats

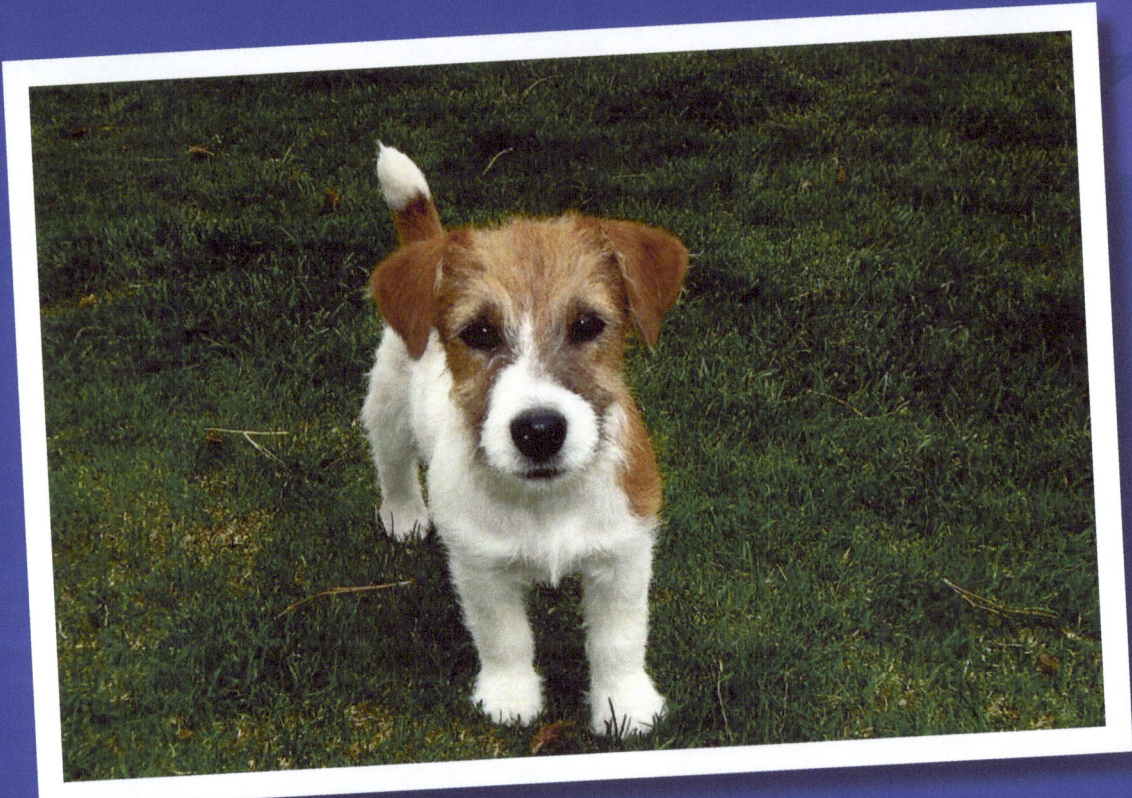

"FRIDAY"

Friday's Favorites
(pumpkin/apple)

Bake at 400 degrees for 18-24 minutes.

In large bowl, add pumpkin puree. Core apples, grate with large hole on cheese grater.

Add grated apples to pumpkin puree. Next add 3 eggs. Mix by hand until well blended.

Add oats to pumpkin mixture slowly, mix by hand. Continue to add until all oats have been mixed in. The dough will be medium to firm.

Roll out ¼ inch thick onto oat-floured surface. Cut with your favorite cookie-cutter shapes.

Place on ungreased cookie sheet. Turn over when it has been ½ the cooking time.

Bake until golden brown.

- **1 cup pumpkin puree**
- **2 large apples, REMOVE seeds**
- **3 eggs**
- **6 cups blended oats**

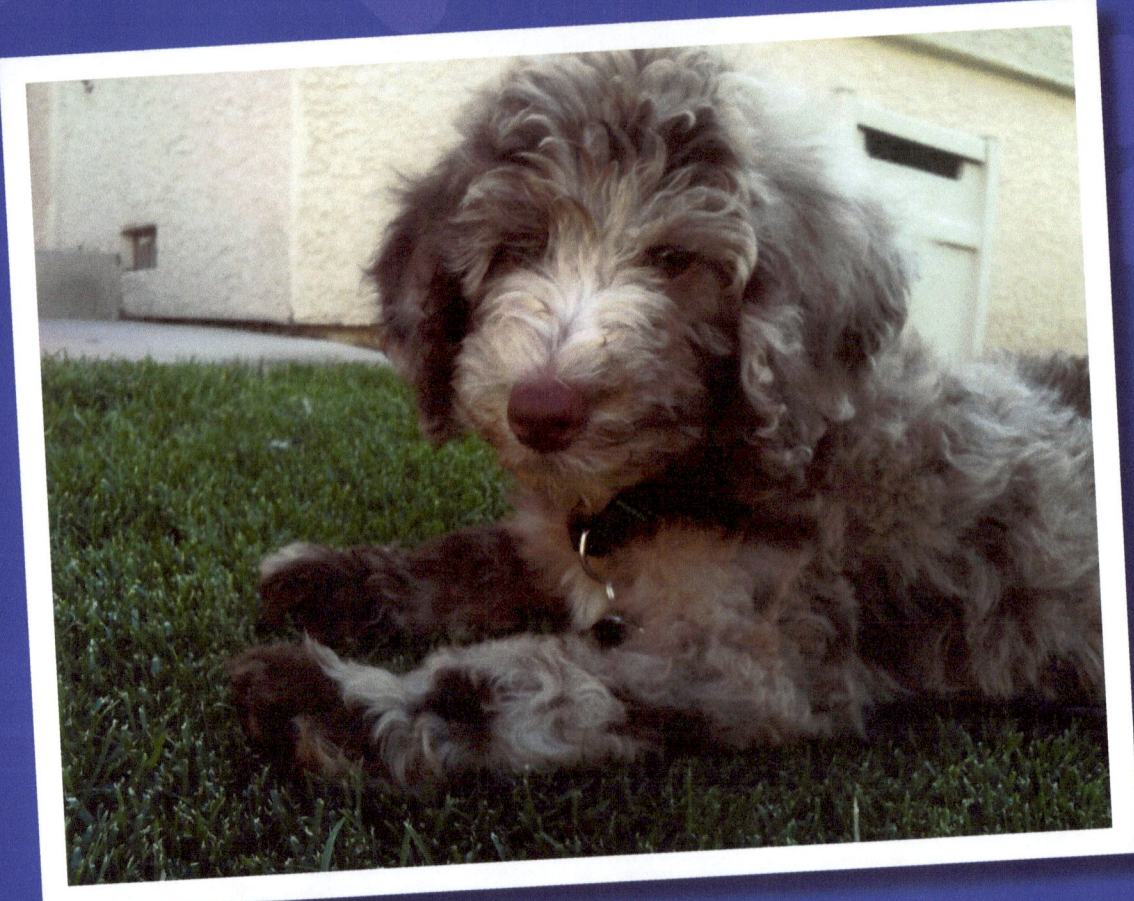

"INDY"

Indiana Banana
(peanut butter/banana)

Bake at 400 degrees for 18-24 minutes.

In large bowl, add peanut butter. Smash bananas with a fork; add to peanut butter.

Put honey in microwave for 5 seconds, add to mix. Now add the 3 eggs.

Mix by hand until well blended.

Add oats to peanut butter mixture slowly, mix by hand.

Continue to add until all oats have been mixed in.

Roll into 1-inch-thick balls. Place on ungreased cookie sheet.

Flatten balls with bottom of a glass or jar. Bake until golden brown.

- 1 cup peanut butter
- 3 bananas
- 2 tablespoons honey
- 3 eggs
- 6 cups blended oats

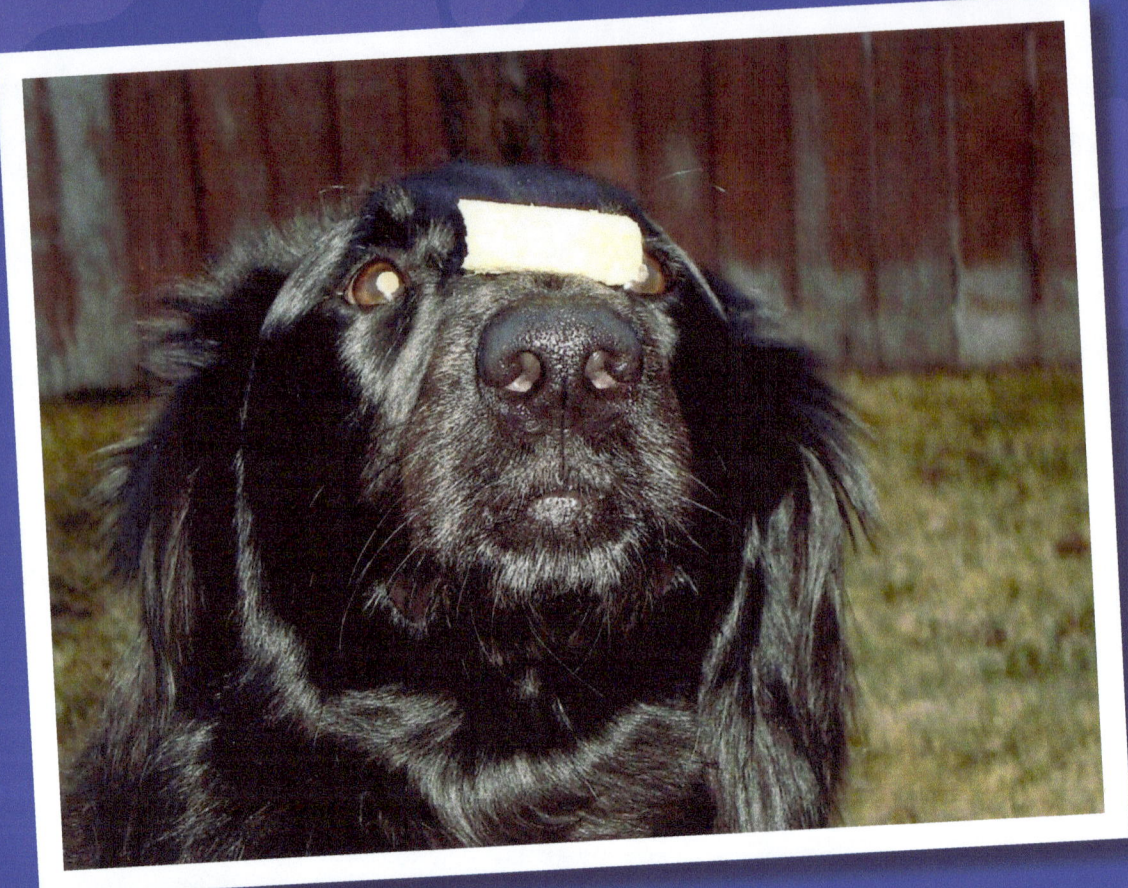

"SHILOH"

Shiloh-Berry
(blueberry)

Bake at 400 degrees for 18-24 minutes.

In large bowl, add pumpkin puree. Place blueberries into a blender and lightly blend;

add blueberries to pumpkin. Put honey in microwave for 5 seconds, add to blueberry mixture.

Next add 3 eggs. Mix by hand until well blended.

Add oats to pumpkin mixture slowly, mix by hand. Continue to add until all oats have been mixed in.

You want the dough medium to firm.

Roll out ¼ inch thick onto oat-floured surface. Cut with your favorite cookie-cutter shapes.

Place on ungreased cookie sheet. Turn over when it has been ½ the cooking time.

Bake until golden brown.

- 1 cup pumpkin puree
- 1 ½ cups blueberries
- 2 tablespoons honey
- 3 eggs
- 6 cups blended oats

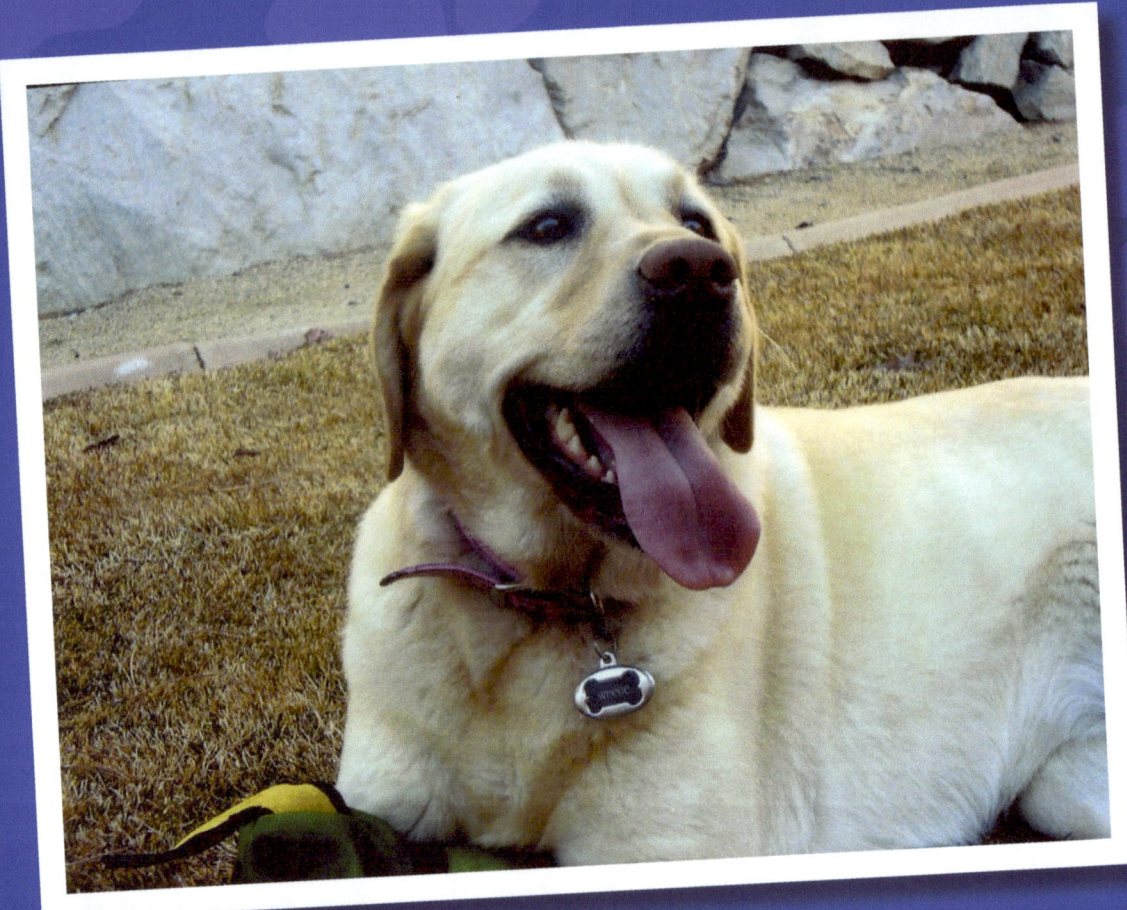

"WINNIE COOPER"

Winnie Waggers
(sweet potato/apple)

Bake at 400 degrees for 18-24 minutes.

In large bowl, add peeled baked sweet potato, smash with a fork. Core apples, grate with large hole on cheese grater. Add grated apples to sweet potato.

Next add 3 eggs and cinnamon. Mix by hand until well blended.

Add oats to sweet potato mixture slowly, mix by hand. Continue to add until all oats have been mixed in. The dough will be medium to firm.

Roll out ¼ inch thick onto oat-floured surface. Cut with your favorite cookie-cutter shapes.

Place on ungreased cookie sheet. Turn over when it has been ½ the cooking time.

Bake until golden brown.

- 1 large baked sweet potato
- 2 medium apples, REMOVE seeds
- 3 eggs
- 2 tablespoons cinnamon
- 6 cups blended oats